Sirtfood D
fami

Tasty, Simple and Healthy Preparations to
Share with all your Beloved Ones

By

Jennifer Young

TABLE OF CONTENTS

INTRODUCTION

Are you looking for a way to change your looks? Do you believe that a diet means to be hungry and be training all the time? If this is your case, this book is for you!

There are tons of miracle diets and low-carbs plans that are always popping up in our phone and, in most of the cases, are not going to be effective for everybody. Through this book, you will learn how to cook and what to buy for adequate meals.

Starting this journey involves new flavours, good meals and the most important part; a whole new world of recipes. If you are looking for a healthy life style and you are done with the veggie/vegan diets, this is the place for you.

Your new life is now one step away. You will discover new ways to help your body have the right performance. We will show you how to:

1. - Help your body to detox.

2. –Burn those extra calories.

3. - Eat tasty and healthy.

4. - Surprise your family with nice and colourful meals.

This is not a regime that is going to make you feel oppressed. You will have lots of options and new flavours every day!

CHAPTER 1 BREAKFAST RECIPES

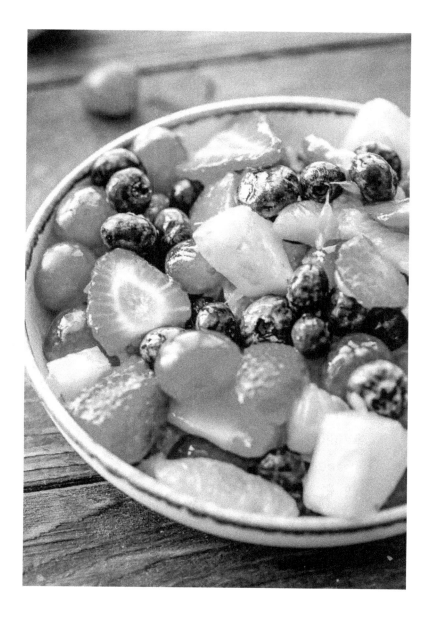

1.1 Fruit Salad

(Ready in about 15 minutes | Servings: 1 | Difficulty: Easy | Course Choice – Breakfast / Snack)

(Nutrition information - Calories:38|Fat:0g|Carbohydrates:18g|Proteins:0g|)

Ingredients

- ½ cup freshly made green tea
- One teaspoon honey
- One orange halved
- One apple, cored and roughly chopped
- Ten red seedless grapes
- Ten blueberries

Instructions

1. Stir the honey into half a cup of green tea. When dissolved, add the juice of half the orange. Leave to cool.
2. Chop the other half of the orange and place in a bowl together with the chopped apple, grapes, and blueberries. Pour over the cooled tea and leave too steep for a few minutes before serving.

1.2 Green Omelet

(Ready in about 15 minutes | Servings: 1 | Difficulty: Easy | Course Choice – Breakfast)

(Nutrition information - Calories:58|Fat:3g|Carbohydrates:8g|Proteins:0g|)

Ingredients

- One teaspoon olive oil

- One shallot, peeled and finely chopped

- Two large eggs, at room temperature

- Handful (20g) rocket leaves

- Small handful (10g) parsley, finely chopped

- Salt and freshly ground black pepper

Instructions

1. In a wide frying pan- heat the oil on medium-low heat and gently fry the shallot for five minutes. Turn the heat up a little bit, and cook for another two minutes.

2. In a bowl or cup, whisk the eggs together well with a fork. Distribute the shallot evenly around the pan before pouring m the eggs. Tip the pan slightly on each side so that the egg is evenly distributed. Cook for a minute or so before lifting the sides of the omelet and letting any runny egg slip into the pan's base. Immediately sprinkle over the rocket leaves and parsley, and season generously with salt and pepper.

3. When cooked, the omelet's top will still be soft but not runny, and the base will be just starting to brown. Tip onto a plate and enjoy straight away.

1.3 High-Fiber Chillas, Buckwheat Oats Indian Pancake

(Ready in about 20 minutes | Servings: 4 | Difficulty: Moderate | Course Choice – Breakfast / Snack)

(Nutrition information - Calories:178|Fat:2.5g|Carbohydrates:28g|Proteins:19.7g|)

Ingredients
For High Fiber Chillas

- ½ cup buckwheat
- ¼ cup low-fat curd
- ¼ cup quick-cooking rolled oats
- One and a ½ teaspoon ginger-green chili paste
- ½ cup grated carrot
- ½ cup chopped spring onions, whites and greens
- Two tablespoons finely chopped coriander
- Salt to taste
- One teaspoon peanut oil for greasing

For Serving with chillas

- Low-Calorie Green Chutney

Instructions

1. To make high-fiber chillas combine the buckwheat, curds, and ½ cup of water in a deep bowl and mix well. Cover with the lid and keep aside for two hours.
2. Blend the mixture to a smooth paste using no water.
3. Transfer the mixture into a deep bowl, add all the remaining ingredients and ¼ cup of water, and mix well.
4. Oil a nonstick tava (griddle) with ¼ teaspoon of oil, and pour a ladleful of the batter, and spread it evenly to make a 125 mm. (5") diameter thin circle, and cook on a medium flame using ¼ teaspoon of oil till both the sides are golden brown.
5. Repeat with the remaining batter to make three more high fiber chillas.
6. Serve the high fiber chillas immediately with low-calorie green chutney.

CHAPTER 2 SNACKS

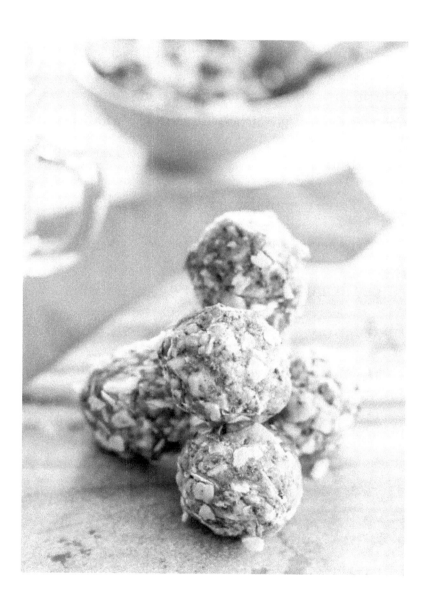

2.1 Date and Walnut Cinnamon Bites

(Ready in about 5 minutes | Servings: 1 | Difficulty: Easy | Course Choice – Breakfast / Snack)

(Nutrition information - Calories:65|Fat:3g|Carbohydrates:18g|Proteins:0g|)

Ingredients

- Three <u>walnut halves</u>

- Three <u>pitted Medjool dates</u>

- <u>Ground Cinnamon</u> to taste

Instructions

1. Carefully cut each walnut half into three slices, then do the same with the dates. Place a slice of walnut on top of each date, dust with cinnamon, and serve.

2.2 Date Bars

(Ready in about 45 minutes | Servings: 8-10 | Difficulty: Moderate | Course Choice –Snack)

(Nutrition information - Calories:238|Fat:9g|Carbohydrates:48g|Proteins:23g |)

Ingredients

Bars

- 200-250 g / 7-9 oz. dates (Medjool dates)

- 65 g / ½ cup chopped almonds

- 65 g / ½ cup chopped walnuts

- 40 g / ¼ cup pumpkin seeds

- 35 g / ¼ cup sunflower seeds

- 30 g / one cup puffed rice

- 25 g / ¼ cup ground flax seeds

- ¼ teaspoon ground cardamom

- 1½ teaspoon vanilla essence

- 30 ml / two tablespoon runny <u>tahini</u>

Topping

- 37 g / three tablespoon <u>coconut oil</u>

- Three tablespoon cocoa powder

- Three tablespoons <u>maple syrup</u> (skip if using 250 g / 9 oz. dates)

- White sesame seeds to garnish

- Sea salt flakes to garnish

Instructions

1. Pit the dates, and soak them in boiling water for 20 minutes. Use 250 g / 9 oz. of dates if you want to use date paste (rather than maple syrup) to sweeten the chocolate layer too.

2. Meanwhile, line a small baking tin (I used a 2lb / 900 g baking tin*) with a piece of baking paper, and preheat the oven to 150° C / 300° F.

3. Mix all the dry ingredients in a large mixing bowl.

4. Place drained dates in a food processor, together with vanilla essence and tahini, and process until smooth. Add 30 ml / two tablespoon (not more.) of boiling water to keep the machine going without getting jammed. Process for five minutes until super smooth and a thick paste is formed. If you are using dates for the chocolate layer, save ¼ cup of the pasta for later.

5. Stir the date/tahini mixture through the nuts and seeds mixture, ensuring it is evenly distributed throughout. You may need to use your hands to do this as the paste is thick.

6. Spread the mixture in the paper-lined baking tin. Press the mixture down sufficiently so that there are no gaps/air pockets and the bars hold together well. Use a piece of baking paper with a flat-bottomed glass on top to pack the mixture better.

7. Bake for about 30-40 minutes; they should be browned, no longer super soft/raw to the touch.

8. Take out of the oven, compress the mixture again using the upside-down glass trick, and then weigh it down with something heavy while the mixture is cooling down. Allow it to cool down completely before cutting or applying the topping.

9. Melt coconut oil on low heat, stir through cocoa powder, and maple syrup

10. Spread the chocolate layer on the cool bars, sprinkle with sesame seeds and salt flakes, and refrigerate until the topping has set.

11. Cut into equal size pieces with a sharp knife. Store the bars in an airtight container.

2.3 Easy Roasted Beet Hummus

(Ready in about an hour| Servings: 2 | Difficulty: Moderate | Course Choice – Sides)

(Nutrition information - Calories:66|Fat:0g|Carbohydrates:28g|Proteins:34g|)

Ingredients

- Two medium beetroots, peeled

- ¾ cup dry chickpeas one can of chickpeas is equivalent

- ¼ cup one lemon, juiced

- Two Tablespoon tahini

- One Tablespoon olive oil

- Two cloves garlic

- ½ teaspoon sea salt

Instructions

1. Cut beets into ½ inch slices and lay on a parchment-covered baking sheet. Roast in the

oven at 400 F for 40-45 minutes, until fork-tender. Set aside to cool.

2. Add all ingredients to a food processor and blend until preferred consistency. Scrape down the sides as needed. If you'd like the consistency to be creamier, add 1-2 Tablespoon more tahini. If you'd like more zest, add more lemon juice.

3. Add hummus to a bowl or plate and garnish with your favorite chips and veggies.

2.4 Easy Vegan Pumpkin Soup

(Ready in about 35 minutes | Servings: 6 | Difficulty: Moderate | Course Choice –Lunch/Dinner)

(Nutrition   information   - Calories:58|Fat:3g|Carbohydrates:8g|Proteins:0g|)

Ingredients

- 2×15ounce cans pumpkin puree

- ½ cup to two tablespoons pure maple syrup two tablespoons

- One cinnamon stick and ¼ teaspoons ground cinnamon

- Two cups low-sodium veggie broth

- One tablespoon chopped fresh rosemary

- One tablespoon smoked paprika

- ¼ teaspoons nutmeg

- ½ tablespoon cayenne omit if avoiding heat

- ½ cup canned coconut milk omit if avoiding coconut

- Four tablespoons vegan butter

- Sea salt and pepper to taste

Instructions

1. Add ½ cup maple syrup and a cinnamon stick to a large pot as the maple syrup starts to boil, then reduce the heat to a simmer, simmer for 5-10 minutes or until the maple syrup thickens. It should thicken to a honey consistency.

2. Slowly stir the canned pumpkin puree into the thickened maple syrup. Add the veggie broth and all other spices to flavor the soup.

3. Cook over medium heat until warmed through, about 10-15 minutes. Stir in one cup of coconut milk (if using). Continue to cook for another five minutes. If the pumpkin soup seems too thick, add more broth or water to thin. Keep over low heat until ready to serve. Remove the cinnamon stick. Once cooled, make pumpkin soup bowls. Serve with toasted bread and vegan butter.

2.5 Edamame and Chili Dip with Crudités

(Ready in about 15 minutes | Servings: 8 | Difficulty: Moderate | Course Choice –Snack)

(Nutrition information - Calories:168|Fat:2g|Carbohydrates:38g|Proteins:50g|)

Ingredients

- 300g <u>frozen soya bean</u>

- 150g <u>low-fat natural yogurt</u>

- One <u>red chili</u>, chopped

- <u>One Lime</u>, juiced

- One <u>garlic clove</u>, crushed

- One <u>red onion</u>, finely chopped

- Handful coriander, chopped

- <u>Halved Radishes</u>, sticks of carrots, celery, and peppers to serve

Instructions

1. Cook the soya beans in boiling salted water for 4 minutes. Drain and cool under cold running water. Blitz with the yogurt, chopped red chili, lime juice, and crushed garlic clove until smooth. Fold in the finely chopped red onion and a handful of chopped coriander. Serve with halved radishes and sticks of carrots, celery, and peppers. The dip will keep covered in the fridge for up to three days.

2.6 Endive Stuffed with Goat Cheese and Walnuts

(Ready in about 40 minutes | Servings: 8 | Difficulty: Moderate | Course Choice –Lunch/Dinner)

(Nutrition information - Calories:168|Fat:3g|Carbohydrates:28g|Proteins:18g|)

Ingredients

- ⅓ cup coarsely chopped walnuts

- Two tablespoons honey, divided

- Cooking spray

- ¼ cup balsamic vinegar

- Three tablespoons orange juice

- Sixteen Belgian endive leaves (about two heads)

- ⅓ cup (one ½ ounces) crumbled goat cheese or blue cheese

- Sixteen small orange sections (about two navel oranges)

- One tablespoon minced fresh chives

- ¼ teaspoon cracked black pepper

Instructions

1. Preheat oven to 350°F.

2. Combine walnuts and one tablespoon honey; spread on a baking sheet coated with cooking spray. Bake at 350°F for 10 minutes, stirring after five minutes.

3. Combine one tablespoon of honey, vinegar, and orange juice in a small saucepan. Bring mixture to a boil over high heat, and cook until reduced to three tablespoons (about five minutes).

4. Fill each endive leaf with one orange section. Top each section with one teaspoon cheese and one teaspoon walnuts; arrange on a plate. Drizzle the vinegar mixture evenly over leaves, and sprinkle evenly with chives and pepper.

2.7 Fresh Saag Paneer

(Ready in about 20 minutes | Servings: 2 | Difficulty: Moderate | Course Choice –Lunch/Dinner)

(Nutrition   information   -
Calories:232|Fat:24g|Carbohydrate:25g|Proteins:34g
|)

Ingredients

- Two teaspoon rapeseed oil
- 200g paneer (cut into cubes)
- Salt and freshly ground black pepper
- One red onion, chopped
- One small thumb (three cm) fresh ginger, peeled, and cut into matchsticks
- One clove garlic, peeled and thinly sliced
- One green chili, deseeded and finely sliced
- 100g cherry tomatoes, halved
- ½ teaspoon ground coriander
- ½ teaspoon ground cumin
- ¼ teaspoons ground turmeric
- ½ teaspoon mild chili powder
- ½ teaspoon salt
- 100g fresh spinach leaves

- Small handful (10g) parsley, chopped
- Small handful (10g) coriander, chopped

Instructions

1. Heat the oil in a wide, lidded frying pan over high heat.
2. Season the paneer generously with salt, and pepper and toss into the pan. Fry for a few minutes until golden, stirring often. Remove from the pan with a slotted spoon and set aside.
3. Reduce the heat and add the onion. Fry for five minutes before adding the ginger, garlic, and chili. Cook for another couple of minutes before adding the cherry tomatoes. Put the lid on the pan, and cook for a further five minutes.
4. Add the spices and salt, then stir. Return the paneer to the pan and stir until coated. Add the spinach to the pan together with the parsley and coriander, and put the lid on. Allow the spinach to wilt for 1-2 minutes, then incorporate into the dish. Serve immediately.

2.8 Garlic Fries

(Ready in about 48 minutes | Servings: 4 | Difficulty: Moderate | Course Choice – Snack)

(Nutrition information - Calories:108|Fat:3g|Carbohydrates:58g|Proteins:0g|)

Ingredients

- Three cloves garlic, minced

- Two tablespoons canola oil

- Three large baking potatoes, 12 ounces each

- ½ teaspoon salt

- One tablespoon finely chopped fresh parsley leaves

Instructions

1. Preheat the oven to 450 degrees F.

2. Heat the garlic and oil in a small saucepan over medium heat for two minutes. Strain the garlic from the oil with a small mesh strainer. Set both garlic and oil aside.

3. Cut the potatoes into ¼-inch sticks. In a large bowl, toss the oil, potatoes, and ½ teaspoon of salt. Spray a baking sheet with cooking spray and spread the potatoes onto it in a single layer. Bake until golden and crisp, about 35 minutes.

4. Remove potatoes from the tray with a metal spatula. Toss with parsley, reserved garlic, and additional salt to taste. Serve immediately.

2.9 Garlic Soup

(Ready in about 35 minutes | Servings: 6 | Difficulty: Moderate | Course Choice – Lunch/Dinner)

(Nutrition information -
Calories:158|Fat:3g|Carbohydrates:38g|Proteins:21g|
)

Ingredients

- Four tablespoons of butter (or ghee)

- Two medium onions (sliced)

- One teaspoon thyme (or two teaspoons fresh)

- One teaspoon dried oregano

- One teaspoon dried basil

- ½ teaspoon salt

- ½ teaspoon black pepper

- ½ batch roasted garlic (the equivalent of 4-5 pounds of roasted garlic)

- One-quart chicken broth

- Two cups canned coconut milk (or other milk of choice)

For Garnish (optional)

- Two tablespoons fresh parsley (minced)

- ¼ cup fresh chives (chopped)

- One fresh lemon (cut into wedges)

Instructions

1. Melt the butter in a large pot and add the sliced onions.

2. Sauté over medium heat, constantly stirring until onions are translucent and golden.

3. Add the herbs and spices, and sauté for an additional two minutes

4. Add the roasted garlic and stir to combine.

5. Add the chicken broth and bring to a simmer.

6. Simmer for 15 minutes.

7. Reduce heat to low and add coconut milk.

8. Use a stainless-steel immersion blender and carefully blend the soup until smooth.

9. If desired, garnish with fresh parsley and chives, and squeeze a lemon wedge over each bowl. Serve warm.

2.10 Garlic Soup with Poached Eggs

(Ready in about 40 minutes | Servings: 4 | Difficulty: Moderate | Course Choice –Lunch/Dinner)

(Nutrition   information   - Calories:178|Fat:3g|Carbohydrates:48g|Proteins:30g|)

Ingredients

- One medium head of garlic, cloves peeled, and thinly sliced

- Three tablespoons olive oil

- Eight (½-inch-thick) baguette slices

- One quarter chicken stock or broth

- ½ teaspoon dried hot red pepper flakes

- Four large eggs

- ½ cup packed small fresh cilantro sprigs

- Four lime wedges

Instructions

1. Cook garlic in oil in a deep 10-inch heavy skillet over low heat, occasionally stirring, until tender, and pale golden, eight to 10 minutes. Transfer garlic to a bowl with a slotted spoon. Add bread slices to skillet, and cook over moderate heat, turning once, until browned, about 4 minutes. Divide toasts among four large soup bowls.

2. Add stock, red pepper flakes, and garlic to skillet, and bring to a simmer.

3. Break one egg into a cup and slide the egg into simmering stock. Repeat with remaining eggs. Poach eggs at a bare simmer until whites are firm, but yolks are still runny, 3 to 4 minutes.

4. Transfer eggs with a slotted spoon to toasts and season with salt. Ladle soup into a bowl and top with cilantro. Serve with lime wedges.

2.11 Garlicky Greens

(Ready in about 20 minutes | Servings: 4 | Difficulty: Moderate | Course Choice —Lunch/Dinner)

(Nutrition information - Calories:123|Fat:1g|Carbohydrates:38g|Proteins:0g|)

Ingredients

- One tablespoon olive oil

- Three shallots, sliced

- Three garlic cloves, sliced

- 150ml hot vegetable stock

- 200g frozen peas

- 600g mixed green vegetables—we used long-stem broccoli, asparagus, and mange tout

- Knob Of Butter

Instructions

1. Heat the oil in a large frying pan and bring a large saucepan of salted water to a boil. Gently

fry the shallots, and garlic for 5-8 minutes, tip in the stock, and peas, then bubble for a few minutes until the peas are cooked.

2. Meanwhile, boil the rest of the vegetables cooking the broccoli and asparagus for a couple of minutes first, then throwing in the final min's mangetout. Drain well, and tip into the pan with the peas. Season, add the butter and mix well.

2.12 Gluten-Free Date Bars

(Ready in about 33 minutes | Servings: 16 | Difficulty: Moderate | Course Choice −Snack)

(Nutrition information - Calories:258|Fat:23g|Carbohydrates:48g|Proteins:8g |)

Ingredients

- One and ½ cup oats (divided)

- ½ cup unsweetened coconut

- 5-6 Medjool dates (4 ounces of pitted dates)

- ½ cup walnuts

- ¼ teaspoons sea salt

- ½ teaspoon baking soda

- One egg

- Two tablespoons ground flax

- ¼ cup coconut oil

Date Layer

- Eighteen Medjool dates (12 ounces of pitted dates)

- One teaspoon lemon juice

- ¼ - ½ teaspoon sea salt (I like ½, but begin with ¼, and add to taste)

Instructions

1. Preheat oven to 325° F.

2. Add one cup of oatmeal to a food processor, a bowl, and process until flour is formed. Add coconut, dates, sea salt, baking soda,

and process until the dates are fully broken up. I find it easiest to process if I break the dates into quarters (if using large Medjools) as I am tossing them into the processor. Last, add the remaining ½ cup of oatmeal and the walnuts, and pulse 8-10 times until the walnuts are chopped but still a bit chunky.

3. The dry ingredients in the food processor add the egg, flax, coconut oil, and pulse until combined. This mixture is the base and the top layer of the bars.

4. Reserve ½ cup of the oatmeal mixture to use as a topping.

5. Line an eight x eight pan with baking paper. Add the oatmeal mixture to the pan and press down into an even layer. I use a pastry roller to pack down the bottom layer.

6. Rinse out the food processor and add date layer ingredients. Pulse 10-15 times until the dates are broken up., then process it for another 3-4 minutes until the dates take on

a light, whipped caramel color. If you soaked the dates, this process should be very easy. If your dates were soft, so you opted not to soak them, and they are not whipping up nicely, you can add 1-2 tablespoons of hot water to help them process smoother.

7. Add the date layer on top of the cookie layer and press down into an even layer. Using a wet hand will keep the layer from sticking and pulling up the cookie layer.

8. Crumble the reserved ½ cup of oatmeal mixture over the top.

9. Bake for 18 minutes.

10. For best results, completely cool before slicing the bars.

2.13 Greek Salad Skewers

(Ready in about 50 minutes |Servings 2 butter cups | Difficulty: Moderate | Course Choice – Brunch / Lunch)

(Nutrition information - Calories:58|Fat:3g|Carbohydrates:8g|Proteins:0g|)

Ingredients

- Two wooden skewers, soaked in water for 30 minutes before use
- Eight large black olives
- Eight cherry tomatoes
- One yellow pepper, cut into eight squares
- ½ red onion, cut in half, and separated into eight pieces
- 100g (about 10cm) cucumber, cut into four slices and halved
- 100g feta, cut into eight cubes

For the dressing

- One tablespoon extra-virgin olive oil
- Juice ½ lemon
- One teaspoon balsamic vinegar
- ½ clove garlic, peeled and crushed
- Few leaves basil, finely chopped (or ½ teaspoon dried mixed herbs to replace basil and oregano)
- Few leaves oregano, finely chopped
- A generous seasoning of salt and freshly ground black pepper

Instructions

1. Thread each skewer with the salad ingredients in the order- olive, tomato, yellow pepper, red onion, cucumber, feta, tomato, olive, yellow pepper, red onion, cucumber, feta.
2. Place all the dressing ingredients in a small bowl and mix them thoroughly. Pour over the skewers.

2.14 Green Fritters

(Ready in about 30 minutes | Servings: 6 | Difficulty: Moderate | Course Choice –Snack)

(Nutrition information - Calories:137|Fat:3g|Carbohydrates:18g|Proteins:32g|)

Ingredients

- 140g zucchinis, grated

- Three medium eggs

- 85g broccoli florets, finely chopped

- Small pack dill, roughly chopped

- Three tablespoons gluten-free flour or rice flour

- Two tablespoons sunflower oil for frying

Instructions

1. Squeeze the zucchinis between your hand to remove any excess moisture, or tip onto a clean

tea towel, and twist it to squeeze out the moisture.

2. Beat the eggs in a bowl, add the broccoli, zucchinis, and most of the dill, and mix. Add the flour, mix again, and season.

3. Heat the oil in a nonstick frying pan. Put a large serving spoon of the mixture in the pan, then add two more spoonfuls, so you have three fritters. Leave for 3-4 minutes on medium heat until golden brown on one side, and soothe lid enough for you to flip over, then flip over, and leave to go golden on the other side. Repeat to make three more fritters (there is no need to add any more oil to the pan after the first batch). Scatter with the remaining dill to serve.

2.15 Green Juice Salad

(Ready in about 12 minutes | Servings: 1 | Difficulty: Easy | Course Choice –Lunch/Brunch)

(Nutrition information -
Calories:48|Fat:2g|Carbohydrates:18g|Proteins:3g|)

Ingredients

- Juice of ½ lemon

- One cm ginger grated

- Salt and pepper to taste

- One tablespoon olive oil

- Two handfuls kale sliced

- One handful rocket (arugula)

- One tablespoon parsley

- Two celery sticks sliced

- ½ green apple sliced

- Six walnut halves

Instructions

1. Put the lemon juice, ginger, salt, pepper, and olive oil in a jam-jar, and shake to combine.

2. Place the kale in a large bowl and pour over the dressing. Massage the dressing into the kale for one minute.

3. Add all the other ingredients, and mix thoroughly.

2.16 Green Mango Salad with Prawns

(Ready in about 20-25 minutes | Servings: 6 | Difficulty: Moderate | Course Choice Lunch/Dinner)

(Nutrition information - Calories:348|Fat:12g|Carbohydrates:38g|Proteins:78g|)

Ingredients

- Two tablespoons <u>lime juice</u>

- One <u>small red chili</u>, seeded and finely chopped

- Two tablespoons <u>fish sauce</u>

- One tablespoon <u>light muscovado sugar</u>

- Three <u>shallots</u>, finely sliced

- 85g roasted salted peanuts, finely chopped

- Two green mangoes or three Granny Smith apples

- Two tablespoons <u>chopped mint</u>

- One tablespoon <u>sunflower oil</u>

- 200g <u>pack raw shell-on headless prawn</u>, peeled but with tail on (or, if you use ready peeled prawns, you need 175g/6oz.)

- Two <u>little gem lettuces</u>

- Two <u>spring onions</u>, shredded

Instructions

1. Mix the lime juice, chili, fish sauce, and sugar in a large bowl. Add the shallots and three-quarters of the peanuts, and mix well. Cover and set aside for up to 4 hours.

2. Peel and coarsely grate the mango or apple, and stir into the mixture along with the mint. Heat the oil in a frying pan or a wok, and add the prawns, and stir fry quickly until evenly pink—about two minutes.

3. Scatter the lettuce leaves on a serving plate, and spoon the salad mixture in the center.

Surround with the prawns, and scatter over the remaining peanuts and spring onions.

2.17 Greens with Herby Lemon Vinaigrette

(Ready in about 20 minutes | Servings: 8 | Difficulty: Moderate | Course Choice – Lunch/Dinner)

(Nutrition information - Calories:238|Fat:0g|Carbohydrates:68g|Proteins:10g |)

Ingredients

- 200g green beans, trimmed

- 250g baby zucchini, halved and quartered lengthways

- 250g peas

- Four tablespoon olive oil

- Two tablespoon lemon juice

- Handful flat-leaf parsley, roughly chopped

- Handful mint leaves, roughly chopped

- One tablespoon snipped chive

Instructions

1. Boil water in a large pan with a steamer attachment and fill a large bowl with ice-cold water. Steam the green beans for 3-4 minutes, the zucchinis for 2-3 minutes, and the peas for two minutes, until everything is just tender. (If you don't have a steamer, just boil the vegetables in boiling salted water for the same times as above.) After cooking, immediately plunge vegetables into the ice-cold water to cool quickly, drain, then pat dry with kitchen paper.

2. For the dressing, whisk together the oil, and lemon juice, stir in the parsley, mint, and chives, then season. Take the dressing and vegetables to the picnic in separate containers, then toss gently together to serve.

2.18 Grilled Asparagus

(Ready in about 30 minutes | Servings: 4 | Difficulty: Moderate | Course Choice –Lunch/Dinner)

(Nutrition information - Calories:78|Fat:0g|Carbohydrates:17g|Proteins:3g|)

Ingredients

- One cup of water

- One pound fresh asparagus, trimmed

- ¼ cup barbecue sauce

Instructions

1. In a large skillet, bring water to a boil; add asparagus. Cover, and cook until crisp-tender, 4-6 minutes; drain and pat dry. Cool slightly.

2. Thread several asparagus spears onto two parallel soaked wooden skewers. Repeat. Grill uncovered over medium heat for two minutes, turning once. Baste with barbecue sauce. Grill two minutes longer, turning and basting once.

2.19 Hearty Vegan Vegetable Stew (Mushrooms and Potatoes)

(Ready in about 40 minutes | Servings: 2 | Difficulty: Moderate | Course Choice –Lunch/Dinner)

(Nutrition information - Calories:178|Fat:0g|Carbohydrates:48g|Proteins:0g|)

Ingredients

- One pack sliced mushrooms trimmed and halved if small or quartered if large

- One small onion chopped

- 2-3 large carrots

- Three garlic cloves minced

- Two tablespoon tomato paste

- Two teaspoons thyme fresh or dried

- Vegetable broth

- One and ¼ water (if needed)

- Five medium potatoes peeled, cut into 1-inch pieces

- One bay leaf

- Two tablespoon lemon juice

- Sea salt and black pepper to taste

- Four tablespoons grapeseed oil

- One tablespoon parsley chopped fresh

Instructions

1. Add grapeseed oil to a large pot over medium heat. Once hot, add onion, carrot, ½ teaspoon sea salt, and cook, often stirring until vegetables are well browned, about 10-12 minutes.

2. Add mushrooms, increase heat to medium-high, stirring continuously until mushroom liquid evaporates, about 10 to 12 minutes.

3. Add garlic, tomato paste, thyme, smoked paprika, and cook until fragrant, about 30 seconds. Scraping up any browned bits. Stir in

veggie broth, water, potatoes, and bay leaf; bring to simmer.

4. Reduce heat to medium-low, partially cover, and cook until stew is thickened and vegetables are tender, 30 to 35 minutes. When complete, discard bay leaf and stir in parsley (or greens of your choice) and lemon juice. Season with sea salt and black pepper to taste and enjoy.

2.20 Hot and Sour Chili Jam with Vegetables

(Ready in about 45 minutes | Servings: 6 | Difficulty: Moderate | Course Choice – Lunch / Dinner / Snack)

(Nutrition information - Calories:148|Fat:3g|Carbohydrates:48g|Proteins:0g|)

Ingredients

- Two garlic cloves

- Three red chilies

- One onion, cut into wedges (skin on)

- Two tablespoons olive oil

- Two tablespoons light muscovado sugar

- Two tablespoons lime juice

- One tablespoon fish sauce

For the vegetables

- 100g young spinach leaves

- 200g French beans, blanched

- Three carrots, cut into thin sticks

- 300g cherry tomato, halved

- Half a cucumber, cut into sticks

Instructions

1. Preheat the oven to 220C/gas 7/fan 200C. Toss the garlic, chilies, and onion in half the oil on a small roasting tin. Roast for 20-25 minutes, until lightly browned. Skin the onion, and garlic, seed the chilies, then blend in a food processor with the remaining oil, sugar, lime juice, and fish sauce until you have a chunky sauce. Add 1-2 tablespoon of water to make it thin to a spoonable consistency if needed.

2. Spoon the jam into a small bowl set on a platter and surround with the vegetables. Ask your guests to help themselves to vegetables, then spoon over the jam.

2.21 Japanese Miso, Kale, and Tofu Soup

(Ready in about 15 minutes | Servings: 4 | Difficulty: Easy | Course Choice – Lunch/Dinner)

(Nutrition information - Calories:178|Fat:3g|Carbohydrates:38g|Proteins15g|)

Ingredients

- 6 ¼ cups vegetable stock
- Six tablespoons white miso paste
- Two garlic cloves finely sliced
- One cm piece fresh ginger peeled and very finely chopped
- One red chili seeded and very finely chopped
- Four spring onions scallions, finely sliced
- 100 g kale trimmed and sliced
- 175 g tofu drained and cut into cubes
- One ½ tablespoon rice vinegar

- 200 g soba noodles 100% buckwheat for gluten-free soup
- Japanese Seven Spice seasoning optional

Instructions

1. Prepare the noodles according to pack instructions, drain, and rinse in cold water. Set aside.

2. Bring the stock to the boil in a medium saucepan.

3. Add the miso paste, garlic, ginger, and chili. Stir to dissolve the miso, lower the heat, and simmer for five minutes.

4. Add the spring onions, kale, tofu, and rice vinegar. Cook until the kale is just tender.

5. Stir in the noodles and serve, sprinkled with some seven-spice seasoning.

CHAPTER 3 LUNCH RECIPES

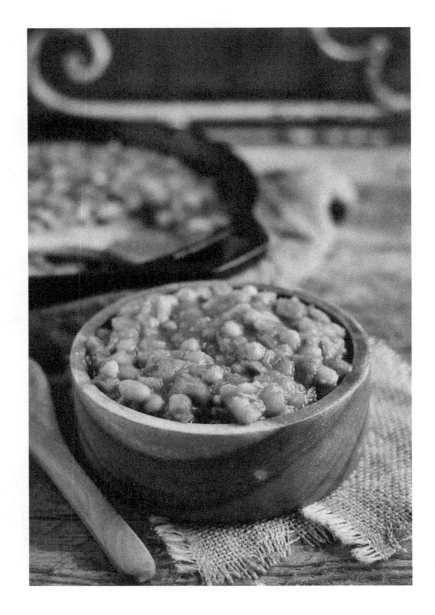

3.1 Easy BBQ Beans

(Ready in about 25 minutes | Servings: 6 | Difficulty: Moderate | Course Choice –Lunch/Dinner)

(Nutrition information - Calories:112|Fat:0g|Carbohydrates:48g|Proteins:0g|)

Ingredients

- One tablespoon olive oil

- One onion, thinly sliced

- Two garlic cloves, chopped

- One tablespoon white or red wine vinegar

- One heaped tablespoon soft brown sugar

- 400g tin pinto beans, drained and rinsed

- 400ml tub passata

- One teaspoon Worcestershire sauce or vegetarian alternative (optional)

- Small bunch coriander, chopped

Instructions

1. Heat the oil in a small pan. Fry onion until starting to brown, then add garlic, and cook for one minute. Add vinegar and sugar, and cook until onions are caramelized. Stir in beans, passata, Worcestershire sauce (if using), seasoning, and simmer for 10-15 minutes until thickened. Stir through coriander and serve.

3.2 Easy Mushroom Pasta with Herbs and Garlic

(Ready in about 25 minutes | Servings: 4 | Difficulty: Moderate | Course Choice – Lunch/Dinner

(Nutrition information -
Calories:208|Fat:9g|Carbohydrates:68g|Proteins:26g
|)

Ingredients

- 8 oz. pasta choice

- 16 oz. mushrooms de-stemmed and sliced

- Three tablespoons dried thyme

- Two garlic cloves minced

- Salt and pepper to taste

- Two tablespoons nutritional yeast add more if you desire

- Two tablespoons dried basil

- Half fresh lemon

Instructions

1. Bring a large pot of water to a boil, and cook pasta according to the package instructions.

2. In a large pan, add the mushrooms, garlic, and few pinches of salt and pepper. Stir occasionally and cook until mushrooms are soft. (About five to 7 minutes)

3. Stir in the cooked pasta along with the dried basil, thyme, and the juice of half a lemon. Serve immediately with nutritional yeast on top.

3.3 Fettuccine Pasta with Capers and Pine Nuts

(Ready in about 15 minutes | Servings: 3 | Difficulty: Moderate | Course Choice-Lunch/Dinner)

(Nutrition information -
Calories:235|Fat:11g|Carbohydrates:48g|Proteins:30g |)

Ingredients

- 9 oz. of gluten-free fettuccine pasta

- 1–2 tablespoons of olive oil

- Dash of sea salt

- ¼ to 1/3 cup Greek yogurt (plain).

- ½ teaspoon minced garlic

- One teaspoon each dried herb mixed

- 1/3 cup capers

- ¼ cup pine nuts

- Two tablespoons fresh basil for topping

- ¼ cup parmesan for topping

- Dash black pepper

Instructions

1. First, boil water, and cook pasta according to instructions. When using gluten-free pasta, be sure to cook el dente and then rinse in cold water after cooking.

2. Return to pot on low and add in olive oil.

3. In a separate bowl, mix your herbs and yogurt.

4. Stir into cooked pasta, and then add in your garlic, and capers, and pine nuts.

5. Stir again and let all the ingredients warm together on a low setting.

6. Add parmesan to the pot or each plate when you serve.

7. Serve and top pasta with fresh basil and cracked black peppers.

3.4 Garlic Chili Prawns with Sesame Noodles

(Ready in about 20 minutes | Servings: 4 | Difficulty: Moderate | Course Choice –Lunch/Dinner)

(Nutrition information - Calories:244|Fat:32g|Carbohydrates:58g|Proteins:86 g|)

Ingredients

- 250g medium egg noodle

- One tablespoon sesame oil, plus extra to serve (optional)

- One tablespoon groundnut oil

- Bunch Spring Onions thinly sliced lengthways

- 300g bag bean sprout

- Four garlic cloves, finely chopped

- One red chili, finely chopped

- 400g raw peeled tiger prawn

- One tablespoon <u>soft brown sugar</u>

- One tablespoon <u>dark soy sauce</u>

Instructions

1. Cook the noodles following pack instructions, then rinse with cold water and drain. Toss with one teaspoon of the sesame oil.

2. Heat two teaspoons of the groundnut oil in a nonstick wok. Stir-fry most of the spring onions and all the bean sprouts for a couple of minutes until tender. Add the noodles and warm through. Stir through the remaining sesame oil, and tip out of the wok onto a serving dish.

3. Carefully wipe out the wok and add the remaining groundnut oil. Toss in the garlic and chili, and cook for 10 seconds. Pop in the prawns and stir-fry for a couple of minutes until they have just turned pink. Stir in the sugar and soy, then bubble until the sugar has melted and prawns are cooked through. Spoon on top of the noodles, and sprinkle with the remaining spring onions. Add an extra drizzle of sesame oil, if you like.

3.5 Garlic Shrimp Pasta in Red Wine Tomato Sauce

(Ready in about 30 minutes | Servings: 4 | Difficulty: Moderate | Course Choice-Lunch/Dinner)

(Nutrition information - Calories:358|Fat:23g|Carbohydrates:68g|Proteins:70 g|)

Ingredients

- One lb. shrimp peeled

- One tablespoon olive oil

- Salt and Pepper for seasoning

- ⅛ teaspoon red pepper flakes

Red Wine Sauce

- One tablespoon olive oil

- ½onion chopped

- Six cloves garlic

- ½cup tomato puree (from the can)

- 28 oz. diced tomatoes (one can)

- ½ cup red wine (such as Chianti)

- ½ cup fresh basil leaves

- One teaspoon Italian seasoning

- ½ teaspoon garlic powder

- ½ teaspoon onion powder

- ½ teaspoon salt

- ¼ teaspoon black pepper

Pasta

- Eight ounces Spaghetti

- ½ cup Parmesan Cheese

Instructions

1. In a large skillet, add olive oil, and heat it over medium-high heat. When the pan is hot, add shrimp and season generously with salt, black pepper, and red pepper flakes.

2. Cook about two minutes, turning shrimp over once, until just cooked through, and then transfer to a large plate.

To make the sauce

1. Add one tablespoon of olive oil in a large skillet over medium heat. Add onion and garlic, and cook garlic is fragrant, and onion is translucent. Add tomato puree and fry for one minute. Stir in crushed tomatoes and add wine. Bring to a boil.

2. Next, add basil, garlic powder, onion powder, Italian seasoning, and salt. Reduce heat to low and simmer while preparing pasta in the next step.

Pasta

1. Cook Spaghetti according to package instructions. Drain and set aside.

Final Assembly

1. Add spaghetti and shrimp into the simmering red wine tomato sauce. Mix well.

2. Serve sprinkled with Parmesan cheese.

3.6 Green Brown Rice

(Ready in about 20 minutes | Servings: 1 | Difficulty: Easy | Course Choice –Lunch/Dinner)

(Nutrition information - Calories:108|Fat:0g|Carbohydrates:38g|Proteins:0g|)

Ingredients

- 150 gm Brown Rice (Cooked)

- One cup Coriander Leaves

- ½ cup Mint Leaves

- 50 gm Onion

- Two pc Ginger

- Two pods Garlic

- Two Green Chilies

- Three Clove

- One pc Cinnamon

- Pepper

- One teaspoon Cumin Seeds

- Two Cardamom

- One teaspoon Oil

- Salt, to taste

Instructions

1. Place coriander leaves, mint leaves, onion, ginger, garlic, green chili, and water in a blender's required amount. Blend them well.

2. Now take some oil in a pan and heat it. Add cumin seeds, cardamom, clove, cinnamon, pepper to it, and sauté.

3. Add onion, the green spice mix to it with some amount of salt.

4. Add cooked brown rice to it, and cook for 10 minutes.

5. Now you can serve you're a bowl of healthy green-brown rice.

3.7 Green Eggs

(Ready in about 20 minutes | Servings: 1-2 | Difficulty: Moderate | Course Choice – Breakfast)

(Nutrition information - Calories:118|Fat:3g|Carbohydrates:18g|Proteins:34g|)

Ingredients

- 1 ½ tablespoon <u>rapeseed oil</u>, plus a splash extra

- Two <u>trimmed leeks</u>, sliced

- Two <u>garlic cloves</u>, sliced

- ½ teaspoon <u>coriander seeds</u>

- ½ teaspoon <u>fennel seeds</u>

- Pinch of <u>chili flakes</u>, plus extra to serve

- 200g <u>spinach</u>

- Two <u>large eggs</u>

- Two tablespoons Greek yogurt

- Squeeze of <u>lemon</u>

Instructions

1. Heat the oil in a large <u>frying pan</u>. Add the leeks, and a pinch of salt, then cook until soft. Add the garlic, coriander, fennel, and chili flakes. Once the seeds begin to crackle, tip in the spinach, and turn down the heat. Stir everything together until the spinach has wilted and reduced, then scrape it over to one side of the <u>pan</u>. Pour a little oil into the pan, crack in the eggs, and fry until cooked to your liking.

2. Stir the yogurt through the spinach mix and season. Pile onto two plates, top with the fried egg, squeeze over a little lemon, and season with black pepper and chili flakes to serve.

3.8 Grilled Mackerel with Soy Lime, and Ginger

(Ready in about 25 minutes | Servings: 2 | Difficulty: Moderate | Course Choice – Lunch/Dinner)

(Nutrition information - Calories:464|Fat:24g|Carbohydrates:58g|Proteins:76 g|)

Ingredients

- 300g mackerel

- 100g jasmine rice

- Four spring onions, sliced

- One red pepper, deseeded, and diced

For the marinade

- One tablespoon low-sodium soy sauce

- Juice One Lime

- Small piece fresh ginger, grated

- One garlic clove, crushed

- Two tablespoons honey

Instructions

1. To make the marinade, mix all the ingredients and pour over the mackerel. Cover and chill for 30 minutes.

2. Heat grill, and put the mackerel, skin-side up, on a baking sheet lined with foil. Grill for five minutes, then turn and baste with the remaining marinade. Grill for five minutes more.

3. Cook the rice following pack instructions, then drain and toss with the spring onions and pepper. Serve with the mackerel.

3.9 Grilled Mackerel with Sweet Soy Glaze

(Ready in about 25 minutes | Servings: 2 | Difficulty: Moderate | Course Choice –Lunch/Dinner)

(Nutrition information - Calories:458|Fat:23g|Carbohydrates:24g|Proteins:88 g|)

Ingredients

- Four mackerel fillets (use our step-by-step guide if filleting from a whole)

- Zest And Juice One Lime, plus extra wedges to serve

- One tablespoon extra-virgin olive oil

- Butter, for greasing

- Steamed Baby Pak Choi to serve

For the sauce

- Two tablespoons soy sauce

- One red chili, deseeded and cut into matchsticks

- Juice One Lime

- Thumb-Sized Piece Ginger, grated

- Two tablespoons muscovado sugar

Instructions

1. Score the mackerel fillets a couple of times on the skin, then lay them in a shallow dish. Sprinkle with the lime zest and juice, and leave to marinate for 5-10 minutes.

2. Place all of the sauce ingredients in a small pan with a splash of water and gradually bring to a simmer. Cook for five minutes to thicken slightly, then remove from the heat, and set aside.

3. Turn the grill to its highest setting, and place the mackerel on an oiled baking tray, skin side up. Sprinkle the fillets with olive oil and some sea salt, then grill for five minutes until the flesh is opaque and cooked through.

4. Divide Pak Choi between plates, lay two mackerel fillets on top, drizzle with the sauce, and serve with a wedge of lime.

3.10 Grilled Marinated Tofu with Citrus Salsa

(Ready in about 1 hour 15 minutes | Servings: 4 | Difficulty: Moderate | Course Choice-Lunch/Dinner)

(Nutrition information - Calories:258|Fat:3g|Carbohydrates:28g|Proteins:16g|)

Ingredients

- One grapefruit

- One orange

- One blood orange

- One ripe but firm avocado (peeled, pitted, and chopped)

- 1-3 red onion (small finely chopped)

- ½ jalapeño (large, or one small-seeded and minced)

- A handful of fresh cilantro leaves (large chopped)

- Sea salt (to taste)

- Black pepper (Freshly ground to taste)

- ½ lime

- 14 ounces firm tofu (one package, organic non-GMO or extra-firm tofu)

- Citrus juice (collected from segmenting the citrus from the salsa recipe above)

- Lime juice (of one lime)

- One tablespoon tamari

- One tablespoon mirin wine (available at Asian markets)

- Maple syrup (Small squeeze of or honey, optional)

- One piece ginger (finely grated and chopped)

Instructions

For the salsa

1. Segment your citrus over a bowl, collecting the juices. Set a bowl with the juices aside.

2. Chop the citrus segments into about ¼-inch pieces. In a separate bowl, combine them with avocado, onion, jalapeno, cilantro, salt, and pepper. Squeeze lime juice on top, and mix gently.

For the Tofu

1. Drain the tofu and wrap it in several layers of paper towels. Place on a plate, cover with another plate, and place a weight on top (a jar filled with water works great). Leave to drain for about 20 minutes.

2. Add lime juice, tamari, mirin, honey, ginger to a bowl with citrus juice from the salsa, and whisk to combine.

3. Unwrap tofu and slice into your preferred shape. Place into a dish that is big enough to hold all of the tofu and the marinade. Pour the marinade over, turning tofu pieces to make sure that they are evenly covered. Leave to marinate for 30 minutes or longer.

4. Grill the tofu for several minutes on each side until golden brown. You can also bake the tofu at 425° for about 20 minutes. Brush with marinade while grilling for an extra bright flavor. Serve with citrus salsa and wilted spinach or other greens.

3.11 Grilled Peppers and Zucchini

(Ready in about 20 minutes | Servings: 4 | Difficulty: Easy | Course Choice –Lunch/Dinner/Sides)

(Nutrition information - Calories:148|Fat:1g|Carbohydrates:28g|Proteins:5g|)

Ingredients

- One medium green pepper, julienned

- One medium sweet red pepper, julienned

- Two medium zucchini, julienned

- One tablespoon butter

- Two teaspoons soy sauce

Instructions

1. Place the vegetables on a double layer of heavy-duty foil (about 18 in. x 15 in.). Dot with butter; drizzle with soy sauce. Fold foil around vegetables, and seal tightly. Grill covered over medium heat for 5-7 minutes on each side or until vegetables are crisp-tender.

3.12 Grilled Vegetable Platter

(Ready in about 50 minutes | Servings: 6 | Difficulty: Moderate | Course Choice – Lunch/Dinner)

(Nutrition information - Calories:238|Fat:0g|Carbohydrates:48g|Proteins:6.3g |)

Ingredients

- ¼ cup olive oil

- Two tablespoons honey

- Four teaspoons balsamic vinegar

- One teaspoon dried oregano

- ½ teaspoon garlic powder

- ⅛ teaspoon pepper

- Dash salt

- One pound fresh asparagus, trimmed

- Three small carrots, cut in half lengthwise

- One large sweet red pepper, cut into 1-inch strips

- One medium yellow summer squash, cut into ½-inch slices

- One medium red onion, cut into wedges

Instructions

1. In a small bowl, whisk the first seven ingredients. Place three tablespoons marinade in a large bowl. Add vegetables; turn to coat. Cover; marinate 1-½ hours at room temperature.

2. Transfer vegetables to a grilling grid; place grid on grill rack. Grill vegetables covered over medium heat until crisp-tender, 8-12 minutes, turning occasionally.

3. Place vegetables on a large serving plate. Drizzle with remaining marinade.

3.13 Grilled wild Salmon with Anchovies, Capers, and Lentils

(Ready in about 50 minutes | Servings: 8 | Difficulty: Moderate | Course Choice-Lunch/Dinner)

(Nutrition information - Calories:358|Fat:13g|Carbohydrates:48g|Proteins:67 g|)

Ingredients

- Four lemons

- Sixteen salted anchovies, rinsed, filleted, and dried

- Extra-virgin olive oil for drizzling

- Eight tablespoon capers, well rinsed

- Six tablespoons finely chopped fresh flat-leaf parsley

- One side of wild salmon, from a 3.5kg/7lb 8oz. fish, cut into 8, 175/6oz. portions

For the lentils

- 300g small brown lentils

- Two garlic cloves, peeled

- Two sprigs of sage (8-10 leaves)

- Six tablespoons extra-virgin olive oil

Instructions

1. Get the lentils ready first. Tip them into a small saucepan, cover with water, and add the garlic and sage. Simmer gently for 15-20 minutes until tender. Drain, discard garlic, and sage season with salt and pepper. Stir in olive oil and set aside.

2. Squeeze the juice of one lemon over anchovies in a bowl, add freshly ground black pepper, and drizzle with olive oil. Mix capers with the parsley in another bowl.

3. Preheat griddle pan until very hot. Season salmon on both sides, then sear, skin-side down (if the pan is very hot, the skin won't stick – this goes for grilling on a barbecue, too). Turn fish over when you see it change color halfway, then sear the other side. This will take 2-3 minutes on each side for rare salmon, but cooking time may vary if fish pieces are very thick.

4. To serve, reheat the lentils and put a large spoonful in the center of warmed plates. Top with the salmon, skin-side up, then scatter anchovies, capers, and parsley on top. Serve with the remaining lemons.

3.14 Healthy Fried Rice

(Ready in about 20 minutes | Servings: 2 | Difficulty: Moderate | Course Choice – Lunch/Dinner)

(Nutrition information - Calories:168|Fat:3g|Carbohydrates:28g|Proteins:32g|)

Ingredients

- One cup cooked cold White or Brown rice

- Two Eggs

- Two cloves garlic finely chopped

- ½ Cup finely chopped Cabbage

- One Carrot finely chopped

- Five Mushrooms sliced

- ¼ cup frozen green peas

- Few florets finely cut broccoli(optional)

- 2–3 spring onions chopped.

- teaspoons sesame oil or vegetable oil(divided)

- One teaspoon crushed black pepper

- ½ teaspoon red chili flakes(optional)

- Salt to taste

- Two teaspoons low sodium soy sauce

Instructions

1. Heat ½ teaspoon of oil in a nonstick pan, and crack open the eggs, allow to sit for a minute, and to use a wooden spatula, start breaking them into small pieces. Fry well and keep them aside.

2. Heat another teaspoon of oil, add in garlic, and fry for few seconds; add all the chopped vegetables, and season with a little salt and half of the crushed pepper.

3. In high flame, allow the vegetables to get fried for a minute until they turn a bit soft but remain crunchy.

4. Reduce the flame to medium, add in the rice, scrambled eggs, and mix well. Increase the flame to high, and fry the mixed rice for one minute, making sure all of the rice is touching the pan's surface.

5. Now make a small well in the middle, pour in the soy sauce and remaining pepper powder, and adjust any salt. Mix the rice well and continue to fry for another two minutes on medium to a high flame by adjusting in between.

6. Add red chili flakes if using and garnish with spring onions before switching off the flame.

7. Serve piping hot with little ketchup if preferred, or eat as it is.

3.15 Herb and Spice Paneer Fritters

(Ready in about 30 minutes | Servings: 12 | Difficulty: Moderate | Course Choice –Snack)

(Nutrition information - Calories:186.4|Fat:16g|Carbohydrates:48g|Proteins:12g|)

Ingredients

- One teaspoon cumin seeds

- 227g pack paneer (Indian cooking cheese, available from supermarkets and Asian grocers), coarsely grated

- Handful coriander sprigs, stems, and leaves finely chopped

- Handful Mint leaves, finely chopped

- One spring onion, finely chopped

- Thumb-size piece ginger, grated

- Two garlic cloves, finely grated or crushed

- Two eggs, beaten

- Two tablespoons <u>plain flour</u>

- <u>Sunflower oil</u> for frying

- <u>Lemon</u> wedges and sweet chili sauce to serve

Instructions

1. Toast the cumin seeds in a large, nonstick frying pan for about one minute, shaking the pan until a shade darker, taking care not to burn. Remove from the heat and place the seeds in a mixing bowl.

2. Add everything else, except the oil, lemon, and chili sauce, to a bowl. Season well and mix very thoroughly. Using wet hands take walnut-size handfuls of the mixture, press into flat little cakes, like fish cakes or patties. They can now be chilled until ready to cook or cooked straight away.

3. Reheat the pan over a medium flame and add enough oil to cover the pan's base. When hot, add the fritters, cook until golden underneath, then turn over, and cook until golden all over. Be careful because they may splutter slightly.

Drain on kitchen paper and keep warm as you cook batches. Serve with lemon wedges and sweet chili sauce.

3.16 Herby Baked Lamb in Tomato Sauce

(Ready in about 4 hours 25 minutes | Servings: 4 | Difficulty: Hard | Course Choice – Lunch/Dinner)

(Nutrition information - Calories:432|Fat:33g|Carbohydrates:58g|Proteins:97.5g|)

Ingredients

- 1.8-2kg shoulder lamb

- Two tablespoons olive oil

- Three oregano sprigs leaves stripped in two

- Three garlic cloves, roughly chopped

- 600ml red wine

- 2 x 400g cans chopped tomatoes

- One tablespoon caster sugar

Instructions

1. Pre-heat the oven to 220C/fan 200C/gas 7.

2. Put the lamb into a large ovenproof dish. Pour the oil into a small food processor with the oregano, rosemary leaves, and garlic, then whizz to a rough paste. Season the paste well, rub all over the lamb, then roast for 20 minutes. Cover, lower the oven to 150C/fan 130C/gas 2, then roast for a further three hrs.

3. Remove the lamb from the oven, and carefully pour off all the fat, leaving any meat juices in the dish if you can. Pour over the wine and tomatoes, poke in the remaining herb sprigs, then return uncovered to the oven for a further 40 minutes. The lamb should now be tender enough to cut with a fork or spoon.

4. Carefully pour or spoon the wine and tomato sauce into another pan, skimming off any fat that rises to the surface, then re-cover the lamb. Let it rest for up to 30 minutes while you roast the potatoes and finish the sauce. Heat the tomato mixture until bubbling, then simmer for 10-15 minutes until thickened and saucy. Season with the sugar and some salt and pepper if it needs it, then pour back around the lamb to serve.

CHAPTER 4 DRINKS

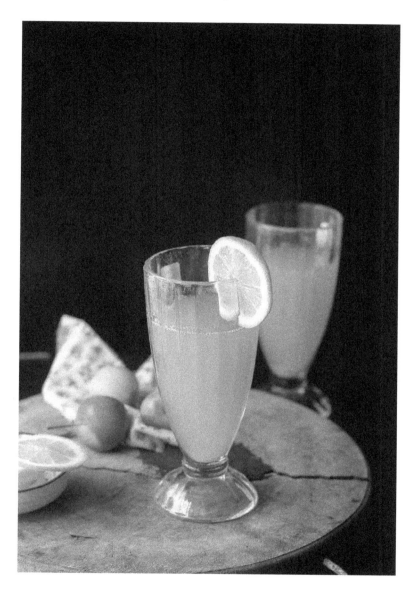

4.1 Grape and Melon Juice

(Ready in about 20 minutes | Servings: 1-2 butter cups | Difficulty: Moderate | Course Choice – Breakfast / Snack)

(Nutrition information - Calories:58|Fat:3g|Carbohydrates:8g|Proteins:0g|)

Ingredients

- ½ cucumber- halved, seeds removed and roughly chopped

4.2 Green Buckwheat Smoothie

(Ready in about 24 Hours| Servings: 1 | Difficulty: Moderate | Course Choice – Breakfast / Snack)

(Nutrition information -
Calories:128|Fat:2g|Carbohydrates:68g|Proteins:7g|)

Ingredients

- One cup baby kale (or baby spinach)

- ½ cup green grapes (frozen)

- ¼ cup carrots

- One tablespoon lemon juice

- ½ cup zucchini (peel it, chop it, and freeze it— makes an awesome thickener for smoothies, a perfect alternative to bananas.)

- ¼ cup buckwheat groats (rinse, soaked overnight in one teaspoon apple cider vinegar)

- One cup hemp milk (or your favorite milk) (freeze in an ice cube tray and thaw 20 minutes before blending to create a slush)

- One tablespoon Baobab powder

Optional

- One handful of fresh mint leaves

- One teaspoon ginger root (peeled, chopped, pressed through a garlic press)

Instructions

1. Soak your buckwheat groats in 3-4 times the amount of water overnight and in the refrigerator. Be sure to add a teaspoon of apple cider vinegar to the water.

2. Soaking this way will break down the natural phytic acid (present on many seeds and grains to protect them as they are grown), and it's important to remove it before we eat it to make it easier to digest.

3. Buy organic zucchini or leave it out - you need organic because this veggie (and like berries) is considered high in insecticide absorption if not grown organically. You must buy it organic.

4. Blend liquids, and leaves first, add zucchini, and the rested blend until smooth.

4.3 Green Smoothie

(Ready in about 5 minutes | Servings: 1 | Difficulty: Easy | Course Choice – Breakfast)

(Nutrition information - Calories:68|Fat:4g|Carbohydrates:28g|Proteins:0g|)

Ingredients

- 250ml <u>milk</u> of your choice (preferred unsweetened almond milk)

- One tablespoon <u>ground flaxseed</u>

- One teaspoon <u>matcha powder</u> (optional)

- Pinch <u>ground cinnamon</u>

- One <u>Medjool date</u>, stoned

- One <u>small ripe banana</u>

- Handful <u>cavolo Nero</u> or spinach

- One tablespoon <u>almond butter</u>

Instructions

1. Pour the milk into a high-speed <u>blender,</u> add the ground flaxseed, matcha powder (if using), and cinnamon. Add the remaining ingredients, then blitz until smooth. Pour into glasses and serve.

4.4 Green Tea Smoothie

(Ready in about 8 minutes | Servings: 2 | Difficulty: Easy | Course Choice – Breakfast / Snack)

(Nutrition information - Calories:58|Fat:3g|Carbohydrates:8g|Proteins:0g|)

Ingredients

- Two ripe bananas
- 250 ml of milk
- Two teaspoons matcha green tea powder
- ½ teaspoon vanilla bean paste (not extract) or a small scrape of the seeds from a vanilla pod
- Six ice cubes
- Two teaspoon honey

Instructions

1. Simply blend all the ingredients in a blender and serve in two glasses.

4.5 Green Tea with Strawberry and Peach

(Ready in about 10 minutes | Servings: 1-2 | Difficulty: Easy | Course Choice – Breakfast / Snack)

(Nutrition information - Calories:68|Fat:1g|Carbohydrates:18g|Proteins:0g|)

Ingredients

- Two teaspoons green whole leaf tea

- Four strawberries, sliced (you don't have to hull them first)

- ½ peach, sliced

Instructions

1. Pour 150ml cold water into a large heatproof jug, then top up with 450ml boiling water. Add the tea leaves and sliced fruit, and leave too steep for two minutes.

2. Meanwhile, fill your teapot with boiling water to warm it. Once the tea has steeped, pour away the water in the teapot, then strain the green tea into the teapot, leaving the fruit and tea leaves behind.

3. You can re-brew this mixture again for another post if you like. Garnish with extra fruit slices if you like.

4.6 Healthy Berry Smoothie

(Ready in about 4-5minutes | Servings: 2 | Difficulty: Easy | Course Choice – Breakfast)

(Nutrition information - Calories:66|Fat:2g|Carbohydrates:13g|Proteins:10g|)

Ingredients

- One handful of arugula or greens of your choice

- One scoop vanilla protein powder

- One tablespoon almond butter

- Two tablespoon ground flaxseeds

- ¼ cup raspberries and blueberries

- ½ cup water add more if needed

Instructions

1. Add all ingredients to a blender and blend until you reach your desired consistency.

4.7 Instant berry banana slush

(Ready in about 5 minutes | Servings: 1-3 | Difficulty: Easy | Course Choice – Breakfast / Snack)

(Nutrition information - Calories:62|Fat:0g|Carbohydrates:28g|Proteins:0g|)

Ingredients

- Two ripe bananas

- 200g frozen berry mix (blackberries, raspberries, and currants)

Instructions

1. Slice the bananas into a bowl and add the frozen berry mix. Blitz with a stick blender to make a block of slushy ice and serve straight away in two glasses with spoons.

CHAPTER 5 DESSERTS

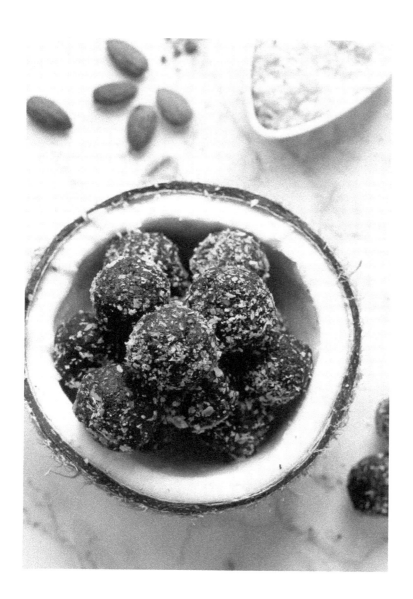

5.1 Healthy Brownie Bites with Medjool Dates

(Ready in about 40 minutes | Servings: 24 | Difficulty: Moderate | Course Choice-Snack)

(Nutrition information - Calories:348|Fat:23g|Carbohydrates:68g|Proteins:54 g|)

Ingredients

- One cup Organic Medjool dates pitted (about 12-14 large ones)

- One cup fresh hot water (for soaking the dates)

- ¾ cup almond flour or any gluten-free flour

- ½ cup Organic Cacao Powder (more for icing)

- ½ teaspoon aluminum-free baking powder

- Three-tablespoon Organic Brown Coconut Sugar

- One tablespoon coconut oil, melted

- Two teaspoons pure vanilla extract

- One large egg

- Pinch or two of sea salt

- A sprinkle cinnamon, optional

- A handful pecans, optional

Instructions

1. Preheat oven to 350 degrees. Line a 9x9 inch pan with parchment paper.

2. Place pitted dates in a medium bowl and pour the hot water over them. Stir and let sit for 10 minutes. Drain the water or reserve for the icing and place the dates in a blender. Blend or pulse the dates until somewhat smooth, making sure all large pieces have been blended. Make sure to scrape the edge of the blender each time you pulse.

3. Add almond flour, cacao powder, baking powder, coconut sugar, melted coconut oil, vanilla, egg, and sea salt in the blender. Blend

until smooth, making sure to scrape the edges of the blender.

4. If adding pecans and cinnamon - place a handful of pecans on top of the brownie mixture and lightly sprinkle the cinnamon.

5. Spread brownie mixture into the baking pan. Bake for 20 minutes. Cool before cutting.

Date Icing for your brownie bites

1. Take your reserved date water and add it to some cacao powder and melted coconut oil until you get the consistency you want for the icing.

2. After the brownies have cooled a bit, pour icing over them. Please note, I did not make the icing for mine.

5.2 Healthy Date Fudge

(Ready in about 1 hour 15 minutes | Servings: 12 | Difficulty: Hard | Course Choice –Snack)

(Nutrition information - Calories:238|Fat:3g|Carbohydrates:58g|Proteins:37g|)

Ingredients

- One cup pitted Medjool date, soaked in warm water for 30 min

- Two tablespoons melted coconut oil

- ½ cup roasted almond butter

- ½ teaspoon pure vanilla extract

- ¼ cup unsweetened cocoa powder

Instructions

1. Remove the pits from dates. Just slice along the center and pop out of the pit.

2. Make sure your dates are pitted and soaked in warm water for about 30 minutes so that they are easier to process. You'll need to melt the coconut oil as well.

3. Next, oil a brownie pan with coconut oil or line it with parchment paper.

4. Combine all ingredients until the consistency is smooth, resembling the appearance of a brownie batter.

5. Combine everything in a food processor.

6. Start with the dates and melted coconut oil, pulsing for about 10 seconds until you have a smooth base to work with, and then add in the other ingredients.

7. Go ahead and taste it. You may want more cocoa powder. To make the fudge even sweeter, add a little honey or maple syrup to taste.

8. Carefully press the mixture in the pan, and top with whatever nuts, seeds, sprinkles, or chocolate chips you desire.

9. Place in freezer for 1 hour or until firm. Cut and serve. Make the squares as big or small as you like. I prefer smaller, two-bite squares.

5.3 Healthy Energy Balls with Medjool Dates

(Ready in about 15 minutes | Servings: 30 | Difficulty: Easy | Course Choice –Snack)

(Nutrition information - Calories:268|Fat:8g|Carbohydrates:46g|Proteins:33g |)

Ingredients

- Eight Medjool dates pits removed

- One cup uncooked old-fashioned oatmeal

- ½ cup ground flax seed

- ⅓ cup unsweetened coconut flakes

- ⅓ cup mini chocolate chips

- One teaspoon vanilla extract

- ½ cup sunflower seed butter (or peanut butter)

Instructions

1. Fill a glass container with very hot water.

2. Add dates to water, cover with plastic wrap, and set aside for 5-10 minutes. This softens the dates and makes them easier to puree, but may not be necessary if dates are very soft.

3. Remove dates from water and place in a small food processor.

4. Add to the food processor about one Tablespoon of the water the dates soaked in.

5. Pulse until smooth, scraping down sides as necessary. Add additional water to thin the consistency of the paste, if desired.

6. Set date "paste" aside.

7. Combine oatmeal, flaxseed, coconut flakes, and chocolate chips in a medium-sized bowl.

8. Add date paste, vanilla extract, and sunflower seed butter to the dry mixture.

9. Stir to combine all of the ingredients.

10. Refrigerate dough for about 15 minutes if possible. (It's not required, but it does make it easier to work with.)

11. Form dough into Tablespoon-size balls.

12. Refrigerate balls in an airtight container.

CONCLUSION

It is amazing how exciting can be the Sirtfood Diet universe and all the new knowledge that you will have. Eating well is not only an esthetical matter; it is crucial for the developing of all the members of your family and provides an adequate care of them.

We live in a globalized world that redefined the concept of food and this is your chance for live alternative lifestyles, where you will have meals that will full fill all your nutrition requirements and will be eco-friendly at the same time.

Fibre, vegetables, balanced meals and water will give you a new perspective in your daily routine. You will have tons of benefits like healthy immune system, mental ability and the only requirement is: start the journey to a better live condition.

Remember that:

1.- It is never too late to start changing a habit.

2.- Vegetables do not have to be prepared in a boring way.

3.- You should have fun experimenting with your own recipes.

Start now and live the experience of having a healthier and simpler life!